I0439973

TREATMENTS FOR

BULIMIA

Treatments For Bulimia

What Is Bulimia And How To Cure Bulimia In 30 Days

Esther Jackson

Copyright © 2013 by Esther Jackson
ISBN-13: 978-1482663921
ISBN-10: 1482663929

All rights reserved. This book or any portion thereof may not be reproduced or used in any manner whatsoever without the express written permission of the publisher except for the use of brief quotations for the purpose of book reviews or articles, without the prior written permission of the publisher.

The information provided in this book is designed to provide helpful information on the subjects discussed. This book is not meant to be used, nor should it be used, to diagnose or treat any medical condition. For diagnosis or treatment of any medical problem, consult your own physician. The publisher and author are not responsible for any specific health or allergy needs that may require medical supervision and are not liable for any damages or negative consequences from any treatment, action, application or preparation, to any person reading or following the information in this book. References are provided for informational purposes only and do not constitute endorsement of any websites or other sources. Readers should be aware that the websites listed in this book may change.

TABLE OF CONTENT

Chapter 1: About Bulimia

Bulimia is a vicious cycle of binging and purging. It brings a tremendous toll on the body and would be even more difficult on the mental well-being of an individual. It is a very difficult condition to deal with. However, this cycle could be broken with the right effort.

An effective bulimia treatment and having the right support would help you develop a healthier relationship with food and help you deal with certain negative feelings. Feelings like tension, shame and guilt are often associated with people suffering from bulimia. In this book, I would share all about this condition in the simplest manner.

Facts To Know About Bulimia

Bulimia Nervosa, or more commonly known simple as bulimia is an eating disorder which is often associated with a person's negative relation towards eating. It is a condition which is related to binge eating and then followed by a frenzied attempt to avoid putting on weight.

If you are someone who is fighting bulimia, life would become an endless battle between that desire to slim down to maintain your thin figure and the mindless obsession to binge eat.

On a subconscious level, you don't prefer to binge. You feel guilty and ashamed about eating after that. However, you buckle under the desire for it. During the average binge, you may take from around 3000 to 5000 calories a single hour. That's a lot.

However, once this stops, you feel terrible and you would look for drastic measures to undo the binge eating. People who have this condition may take Ex-Lax, going on excessive running/exercises or may force themselves to vomit. And as time passes, they would feel more and more out of control. They feel like they can't control their behaviour at all.

It is very important to note that although many people associate bulimia with purging, it isn't necessary such. There are other acts of self-torture as well. This includes doing away with food from your body by throwing up or using excessive laxatives, enemas or diuretics. Different patients make up for the binge differently - from fasting, excessive working out and going on crash diets. These are all general tendencies of the bulimia patients.

Are You Someone With Bulimia?

Many people constantly wonder if they have bulimia. They feel like they have some of the tendencies but find it hard to decide by themselves if they have this condition. This is easy. You can ask yourself these questions.

The more you answer with 'yes' the higher the probability of you suffering from bulimia or have a different eating disorder.

These questions include:

- Does food and dieting play a major role in your life?

- Are you constantly worried about your body and weight?
- Do you have this fear that once you start eating, you can't quit?
- Do you feel ashamed, guilty or dejected when you start eating?
- Have you eaten till you feel sick?
- Do you constantly purge or take laxatives to check your weight?

The sufferer of bulimia nervosa would commonly not show any dramatic weight loss compared to those sufferers of anorexia nervosa. Most of them may actually look very healthy. However, they are not. Bulimia is often a mental condition where the sufferer feels out of control.

Among teenagers, between 2.5 to 4% of them have either of these condition - anorexia nervosa or bulimia nervosa. The Eating Disorder Centre (EDC) reports that this is a very high number and has to be looked deeply into.

Those sufferers who have bulimia are often known as bulimics. Their behaviours involve gorging and they have various methods of purging which happen constantly over a long period of time. As such, there are a few complications which may arise.

Among the complications which could arise include:

- Electrolyte Imbalance

- Other Damages To The Throat Or Esophagus
- Stomach Issues, Including stomach rupture
- Ulcer and Pancreatitis
- Laxative addiction
- Death
- Other heart issues including coronary failure

Bulimia nervosa is a condition which tends to run in families. This may be the result from certain reasons, from genetics to environment issues. It is common sense because the parents would normally influence the children with how they look from a young age.

Besides that, bulimia is also linked to depression and obsessive compulsive disorder (OCD).

Like other eating disorders, the bulimia nervosa treatment is multifaceted in order to deal with the different causes which affect it and the problems associated with it.

Among the crucial things that need to be done include educating them about nutrition and alteration of their behaviour. This includes changing their eating habits, creating the exercise habit, resolving their interpersonal problems and addressing any mood problems. These are all important in controlling the bulimia condition.

Alyssa The Bulimic

Again, Alyssa is on a liquid diet. She has told herself that she would stick by it and that she won't buckle under her cravings this time. However, she doesn't have the resolve to do it and all she thinks about is food. Finally she decides to give in to those impulses to binge. She can't control herself any longer.

She would grab a pint of ice cream from the freezer and gulp it down in a few minutes. From there, she would look to eat just about anything from the kitchen. Following an hour of binge eating, she feels so full that she is going to explode.

She feels disgusted with herself and panic by the thousands of calories she has taken. She goes to the bath tub to throw up by inserting her fingers in her mouth.

She goes to her weight scale after vomiting to check that she hasn't put on any weight. She tells herself, "Tomorrow I will start again." But she never does as she goes through this torturous cycle again.

This is a condition that bulimics face. It is a mental association with food that needs to be fixed.

Chapter 2: Understanding Bulimia Cycles and Symptoms

The binging and purging cycle is a difficult one to endure. It goes like this: Dieting would trigger the bulimia's destructive cycle of binge eating and purging.

This difficulty arises because the stricter and more rigid the diet is, there is an increased possibility that the sufferer would think about food. He or she would be constantly haunted and preoccupied by eating. When starving yourself, the body would react with more powerful cravings. That is the way the body asks for more sustenance.

How The Bulimia Process Works

As the hunger, stress and desire for eating get more; there a general compulsion to eat more and more. For example, if a bulimic look to lose weight and decides not to eat pasta, there is even more compulsion to eat this. It is considered your 'taboo' food.

With this all-or-nothing mentality, you may feel that any let off in your diet as a complete failure. Once you consume a small spoon of pasta, you may feel completely like a failure. There is a feeling that since you have already failed, you might as well go all out.

However, the relief that comes from binge eating is transitory. Suddenly after that, the guilt and self-loathing would come in. As such, the sufferer would purge to make up for gorging and to regain control.

Purging simply reinforces binge eating. You may tell yourself to launch into a fresh diet and that this is the last time that you fail to follow it. There is a voice at the back of your brain which tells you that you are able to throw up or use laxatives if you fail again. What you may not realize is that purging doesn't come close to wiping the slate clean follow your binge.

Purging Wouldn't Help You Lose Weight

This is a belief that many people with bulimia have - that purging would help them lose calories. However, this is totally false. That is the reason why many people who suffer from bulimia would actually end up gaining weight over a period of time.

Vomiting may help only with less than half of the calories consumed at best. For most situations, these are much less. This is because calories are absorbed the moment you place food into your mouth.

The other method which many bulimics use is through laxatives and diuretic drugs.

Even that, they are even less effective. Laxatives may only do away with around 10% of the calories consumed while diuretics may not even do anything. You may weight lesser after taking them, but the weight loss is not real. It is simply due to water loss in your body.

Signs And Symptoms

If you have a long history of bulimia, you have probably experience all the signs of binging and purging habits. It is only human to be ashamed about the difficult time in controlling yourself with the food you eat. As such, you would most probably binge alone.

When consuming doughnuts, you would replace them so that your loved ones won't notice this tendency. Other signs may be when you purchase your food for a binge and head to several markets so that people won't realize.

Although it may be hard for those who aren't close to you to detect, those who are closest to you might have sense that something isn't right through your behaviour. These are among the common signs and symptoms of bulimia.

These are the sign and symptoms of binge eating:

- **No Visible Weight Gain**. Eating incredibly large amount of food but no visible weight gain.
- **Lack Of Control Over Eating**. They may find it difficult to stop eating and they may even eat until they feel physically uncomfortable and painful.
- **Secretive Eating**. They may go to the kitchen once everyone has slept or going out alone on food runs. They may also decide to eat in privacy.

- **Disappearing Food**. Certain food may disappear from the fridge suddenly. Many empty wrappers in the trash or hidden junk food are also common tendency.

- **Constant Changing Between Overeating And Fasting**. These patients rarely consume standard meals. They either eats a lot at one go or not eat at all for a certain period.

These are the common signs and symptoms of purging:

- **Unreasonable Exercising**. Sufferers would work out strenuously. Worst still, they may exercise right after they eat. They may also indulge in distinctive activities which are high intensity calorie burners. This includes activities like running or aerobics.

- **Scent Of Vomit**. When you go to the sufferer's bathroom, you may be able to smell vomit. They may try to cover up the smell with mouthwash (if they themselves smell), perfume or air fresheners.

- **Immediate Baths**. Going to the baths immediately after meals. The sufferers would often disappear the moment they take their meals or head to the bath to throw up. They may run the water to cover up the sounds of their vomiting.

- **Utilize Certain Pills** to induce vomiting. They may use laxatives, diuretics or enemas after eating. They may take diet pills to curtail appetite or use the sauna to sweat out their weight.

These are the common physical signs and symptoms when someone has bulimia:

- **Frequent Weight Variation** - Your weight may waver by around ten pounds or more due to this constant binging and purging.
- **Calluses or scars on the knuckles and hands.** This is because these sufferers tend to stick their fingers down the throat to force vomiting.
- **Swollen cheeks** due to constant vomiting.
- **Discoloured teeth**. This is due to the exposure to stomach acid when they

vomit. Their teeth may look yellow or ragged.

People who suffer from this condition are not necessarily skinny. Bulimia isn't the same with anorexia. People with bulimia would have normal weight or probably even overweight. Being skinny while purging may indicate that they have some sort of anorexia condition.

These signs are important in determining if you or your loved ones have this condition. If you find it hard to decide by yourself, you can ask your loved ones to check on you. They would be able to know better if you show these signs.

Chapter 3: How Bulimia Affects A Bulimic

For someone living with bulimia, they are putting their body and life at risk. Among the most life-threatening side effect from bulimia is dehydration due to purging. Unfortunately, this is a very common condition among bulimics.

Electrolyte imbalances may happen in the body. They are caused by laxatives, throwing up and diuretics. This is most generally in the form of low potassium levels. When someone has low potassium levels, it would trigger many symptoms which range from lethargy and cloudy thinking. This may also cause irregular heartbeats and probably death. If you have a chronically low level of potassium, this could even result in kidney failure.

The Dangers Of Bulimia

Although there are several effects from bulimia, among the most obvious ones are how it could impact your teeth and mouth. When the sufferers purge by regurgitation, it would bring up the acid from their stomach to the esophagus and slowly into their mouths. The acid would then wear out the natural teeth enamel.

Other bulimia effects would also include sores, cavities and gum infections. The sufferer's esophagus would also get irritated as the travelling stomach acids which are travelling towards the mouth may produce heartburn.

Other sufferers who purge using certain laxative methods would frequently become constipated. They would have atypical bowel movements and this would get truly hard for them. Another common effect of bulimia is that it would lead to malnutrition and an unhealthy body over a period of time.

Other bulimia effects on the body also include chronic kidney issues because of vitamin and mineral deficiencies. When bulimia is frequent, this could even lead to kidney failure. They may become dehydrated and this would lower your body's electrolytes. This would cause irregular heartbeats or certain heart issues.

Bulimia isn't just a physical problem but also something which affect heavily on a person's psychology. Those people who have a lack of self-esteem or self-assurance may have depression if not dealt with properly. Depression is a condition which affects a person's entire life. As such, this condition wouldn't just affect the sufferer but would affect the people close to them as well.

If you or someone you happen to know has this condition, you should seek all the required information to begin getting help. Different kinds of sufferers would require treatments. However, you wouldn't know what you need until you look for professional help. Those who develop this disorder are normally perfectionists who are very eager to please other people.

Anyone who has bulimia requires all the help and support that they can have. They need to seek professional help to turn their lives around immediately and building some self-esteem.

Despite all those information that I have shared in the past few chapters, there are still additional complications and adverse effects that bulimia can have on you. They may include:

- Feeling dizzy and weak
- Broken blood vessels in the eyes
- Constant sore throat
- Hand and feet swell
- Abdominal pain
- Weight gain
- Acid reflux
- Stomach ulcers
- Chronic constipation from laxative abuse

About Ipecac Syrup

Ipecac syrup is a type of medication which is used to induce regurgitation. If you are using it after a binge, be very cautious. The regular usage of ipecac syrup is very deadly. Ipecac would build up in your body over time and sooner or later, it would lead to heart damage and a sudden cardiac arrest.

I can't stress this enough, but the side effects of bulimia are internal. You would have organ problems like malnutrition due to the body not soaking enough nutrients, irregular heartbeat and feeling of overall weakness.

The physical effects of bulimia are simply on the surface compared to the psychological damages. Research being done has proved that bulimics are often perfectionist. They let a great deal of their behaviour be controlled by the need to please others.

People who suffer from bulimia are also known to feel depressed sometimes. This is often due to a chemical imbalance in the brain. This isn't a simple disorder as it may even take control of the person's entire life.

You must never take this condition lightly. It may be difficult to observe some of the side effects of this disorder but it this condition is left alone and neglected, it would lead to many other more severe medical issues. In even more serious condition, this would also lead to death.

Bulimia is a condition that has caused the death to thousands of teenagers and even grownups. This shows that even if you are older, you may not be totally comfortable with your image.

Therefore, it is important to look closely and see if you or your loved ones have those bulimia side effects. Try to offer them all the help and support.

If you are indeed someone who suffers from bulimia, don't be afraid to ask for somebody's help, especially those who are closest to you. Better still, ask for professional advice.

Chapter 4: The Cause Of Bulimia

It is very difficult to find a single cause of bulimia. Low self-esteem and extreme worrying about the weight and body image play a very huge role but there are other additional contributing causes.

In most circumstances, people who suffer from bulimia or any other eating disorders have big trouble in managing their emotions in a sound manner. Eating becomes an emotional release for them. As such, you shouldn't be surprised when these people binge and purge when they feel blue, angry or anxious. Without a doubt, bulimia is an extremely complex emotional problem. Among the major causes or risk factors for bulimia includes:

- **Extreme Low Self-Esteem**. People who think of themselves as worthless, unattractive or useless are at high risk of bulimia. There are several things which contribute to this, including perfectionism, depression, childhood abuse and a home environment which was critical.

- **Poor Body Image**. There is a tendency in our culture to put a priority on being thin and beautiful. As such, this leads to an extremely dissatisfying view on our body. This is especially apparent in young women who are constantly bombarded with constant images of an unrealistic ideal of their physical body. This unrealistic idealization on slenderness has resulted in a poor body image and unrealistic measurement on beauty and success. From television, movies and magazines; everywhere you see people emphasizing on having that lean body. They put a priority on having a slender body more than anything else.

- **Dissatisfaction with their body and feeling fat**. This drive for slenderness led many women to become too concerned about their looks. Research has even showed that many people who are of normal weight or even skinny are extremely dissatisfied with their body. As such, they develop inappropriate behaviour to control their food consumption.

- **Adolescent Pressure**. The American Association of University Women made a discovery that adolescent girls trust that how they look would play an important role in their worth and their body image play a huge part in their sense of self.

- **Personality Trait**. Many people with bulimia share certain personality traits. This includes a feeling of helplessness, low self-respect and constantly fearful about being fat. Those who suffer from bulimia have eating behaviours as a method of handling tension.

- **Trauma or Ill-Treatment by Others**. Those who have bulimia may have probable incidence of sexual abuse. Those people with bulimia are also have a higher probability of parents with a problem with substance abuse or other psychological disorder.

- **Runs In Family**. According to multiple researches on bulimia, it seems that it runs in families, with females most heavily affected. Similarly, there is growing evidence to suggest that a girl's immediate social environment which affects her body image. This includes how her family and friends view their body as well. They may have put a tremendous importance of thinness and looking good. For example, if your family puts a lot of discussion on looking good and be thin, then it is very normal to feel that you have to be thin as well.

- **Being Teased By Close Ones**. If you find yourself constantly being teased by your friends or loved ones regarding low self-esteem and constant eating disturbances in young girls, you would be influenced without a doubt. Studies on girls who live in such families that are rigid and place a strong emphasis on physical attractiveness are at a heavier risk for developing bad eating behaviours.

- **Profession Pressure**. Besides, individuals who have certain profession like modelling, dancing, wrestling or gymnastics are more susceptible to this condition.

- **Major Life Changes**. Bulimia is also triggered when there are major changes in a person's life. This includes puberty, the collapse of an intimate relationship or moving away for college. Normally, a person binge and purges as a method of coping with the tension.

- **Biochemistry Influences**. Studies have found that there is a strong correlation between biological factors that are most common among those with clinical depression and the development of bulimia. Stress hormones are elevated in people who have bulimia while neurotransmitters, like serotonin may not function well.

According to a thorough research of over 15,000 adolescents, youngsters as young as 10 years old are inducing regurgitation in order to lose weight. In fact, purging was a serious issue among those who are aged 10-12 years of age. In a staggering statistic, more boys are affected than girls, according to this report.

The study also trailed a person's sleeping patterns, daily activities and diet and came to a conclusion. It concluded that self-induced regurgitation was very prevalent among teenagers who are trying to slim down.

It also noted that living a sedentary lifestyle, having insufficient sleep and bad eating habits would also contribute significantly to this behaviour.

According to the study as well, teenagers who had more than two hours of daily screen time (from computers or television) tend to utilize purging more than those who have less than two hours.

It also found out that paediatric obesity rates have done up around three times in industrialised nations. It is of no surprise that purging is a very common weight control method.

The researchers have numerous hypotheses for the higher rates of purging among the boys compared to the girls. This is because boys are more commonly associated with obesity compared to girls. However, most of them are totally unaware that their weight control behaviour is extremely unhealthy.

This alarming rate of eating disorder among teenagers has sent out a tremendous warning to schools about the importance of early intervention. Another important point is that while most attention is on female sufferers of bulimia, increased attention should also be given to males who suffer from this problem.

Chapter 5: Bulimia Deficiencies and Dealing With Them

During puberty and adolescence, it is a very turbulent time if these group of people under-eat. It is very important that adolescents eat well during this period as their body is still growing.

Through this period of time, your body is developing rapidly and it calls for a minimum of 2500 high quality calories in a single day. Many girls, in their ignorance, choose to diet and take less than 1000 calories each day. This starving diet would quickly develop into compulsive eating for bulimics.

Like anorexia, bulimia is often found because there is an over-emphasis on a diet mind-set. Alyssa's story was a common but typically unhappy one. She has a healthy and strong body. She never dieted in her life but she attended flight attendant training and observed that most of the trainees were steady dieters.

During the training, she didn't eat nutritious food nor had her usual exercises. As such, she found herself putting a little weight. Concerned about her appearances, she started skipping meals. Very soon, her starving slowly turned into binging and purging. By the time she finished her course, which is only three months later, she has acquired unbearable cravings for sweet stuffs. However, she was binging and purging around four to six times a week.

Nevertheless, with the use of supplements or other treatment, many bulimic women like Alyssa could return to their original weight and health.

It is extremely easy to become bulimic because of the environment. The main reason that both binging and vomiting would trigger a wave of very powerful brain chemicals called the endorphins.

The release of endorphins, which is a form of organic heroin-like brain chemicals, would help build a powerful obsession that bulimics would need to battle. The moment we start developing false thoughts about how much we ought to weight and start dieting, we create the first step of developing an eating disorder, similarly to what Alyssa did.

A great number of women and men are pressured by the dieting mind-set to a point where it becomes very dangerous. They have lost their appetites and weight. They are not driven by eating healthy food but rather unhealthy food to satisfy their short term cravings like cheeseburger.

In another case, Debra started her first ever diet at the tender age of only thirteen. By then, she had developed the major symptoms of anorexia. She was constantly sick with colds, was too weak to exercise and lose her menstruation.

She stopped meeting up with her friends and stayed at home. She started having mood swings which include insomnia, having a bad temper and hysteria. Very soon, her diet became more and more extreme. She started taking just one apple a day.

Debra's' symptoms cause her to have terrible malnutrition problem. Many of the people with anorexia actually get high when they starve. Anorexia also sparks off a certain high that opiates like heroin given to drug addicts.

Anorexic starvation is similar to bulimic regurgitation and binging. It is a very traumatic experience which would stimulate a survival of the fittest mechanism. The release of endorphins would also allow us to go through pleasure, kill the pain from starvation and ease tension.

Anorexics would constantly defend their refusal to eat based on potent biochemical reasons. Meanwhile, bulimics binge and would turn away from keeping the food down similarly for the same reasons. Their obsessive behaviour is caused by nutritional deficiencies, which we would address in the next few chapters.

How Nutritional Deficiency Would Lead To More Eating Disorders

We would look at how two vitamin and mineral deficiencies are generally caused by low caloric dieting. We would also trace their course on how they would activate the eating disorder symptoms.

When you are depleted by under-eating, the Vitamin B1 in your body would be lesser. This Vitamin is something that your body can't make and you could only get them from foods, mainly whole foods that many dieters stop eating. This includes food like whole grains, seeds, meats, beans and veggies.

Among the general symptoms of Vitamin B1 deficiency includes:

- Depression
- Irritation
- Fatigue
- Sleep Disturbance
- Chest Pain
- Tension
- Abdominal Soreness
- Loss Of Appetite
- Loss of Weight

At some point of a bulimic's diet, their B1 levels may have dropped to a danger zone. They might still be the same person, but you would want day have enough

Vitamin B1 and one day you might not. As such, the anorexia symptoms would erupt quickly without warning. This may include sores on the skins or a sudden loss of appetite.

When Vitamin B1 deficiency happens and defeats a person's appetite, the sufferer would eat lesser especially when they are already dieting. Suddenly, dieting becomes simpler and you are not fighting common place appetite any longer. You would simply lose it the moment you lose too much Vitamin B1 from dieting.

You can't decide on what you would lose in a diet. It isn't that we simply lose body fat. We also lose bone density, muscles and brain tissue as well. According to brain scans, anorexics have void spaces which show up when they suffer a loss in brain weight.

Zinc is another mineral which is hard to come by in foods. They are normally found in food like egg yolk, red meat and sunflower seeds. However, these foods are high in fat and are most probably not in a dieter's meal. As such, those who diet are always at the risk of zinc deficiency. According to eating specialists, a great deal of overeaters and bulimics has this tendency of being zinc deficient.

Zinc is the second most abundant trace element in the body and is extremely influential in the proper functioning of the body. If you don't have enough zinc, the body may only register extreme saltiness, sweetness or spiciness as having any sort of taste.

Very often, we all complain that those simple and healthy foods are unappetizing. This is also the same problem that anorexics face.

When faced with zinc deficiency, they would normally develop other symptoms like sluggishness, retarded growth and a disruption in their sexual development as well.

In a five year study conducted, it is reported that there is a tremendous finding that increases the recovery rate for anorexia patients. Those patients were simply given zinc supplementation. It results in weight gain, better outlook and increased bodily function.

It is extremely important that teens have an adequate amount of zinc in their body. This is because when they are in puberty, their reproductive development is at its peak. Zinc is very important to ensure the reproductive function as well as immune roles, mental lucidity and appetite.

If a teenager cuts down the zinc and other minerals supply from its diet at the nutrient-demanding growth stage, not only would the appetite disappear but a teenage girl's menstruation may fizzle out together with her mental function.

That is why an eating disorder can be so dangerous. For teenage boys or men, zinc is a chief ingredient in sperm production and protects against prostates jobs and feeble immunity.

Brain Issues From Protein Malnutrition

As the brain activeness shrink from dieting, the brain's mental and emotional stableness may falter and even conk out. There are several brain chemistry deficiency symptoms including depression, anxiety, obsessiveness and low self-esteem. Those who are known to diet always or have eating disorders would suffer from constant mood swings causes primarily from protein malnutrition.

The brain chemicals which prescribe your moods are gained from amino acids in protein foods. Even those people who don't diet tend not to eat enough protein and would suffer from low-protein brain issues.

About Tryptophan Depletion

The most familiar of the brain's four chief mood regulators, the Serotonin, is made from aminoalkanoic acid L-tryptophan. As there are only few foods which bear elevated amounts of tryptophan, it is one of the first nutrients which you may lose while on a diet.

A study has showed that levels of serotonin may drop too low within 7 hours of tryptophan depletion. We can follow this individual essential protein (9 altogether) as it becomes more depleted by dieting. This depletion may turn you towards driven eating, depression, anorexia and bulimia.

When the levels of serotonin fall, so do our feelings of esteem. These feelings are mainly the result of not eating those protein foods which sustain our serotonin levels. As their serotonin dependent self-esteem drops, girls would tend to diet more. However, they fail to understand that they would never be skinny enough to satisfy their brain which is starving for nutrients. Without a doubt, extreme dieting is the worst way to raise self-esteem. The brain would only deteriorate more and become more critical as it starves.

The moment tryptophan deficiency induces the drop in serotonin levels, you may become obsessed by thoughts which you simply can't switch off or certain chronic behaviours which you simply can't stop. The moment this rigid behaviour pattern comes out during dieting, the sensitivity towards eating disorder is complete.

Many people are obsessed with calorie counting and this makes them feel worst over time. They tell themselves to eat less. As they eat lesser and lesser, their serotonin levels decline even further. This increases the person's compulsion to under-eat. As their levels of zinc and Vitamin B drop too, their appetite would be lost and this enhances their chances for anorexia.

Tryptophan And Bulimia

For certain unusual reasons which are hard to comprehend, some dieters have serotonin levels which drop but don't lose their appetite. They may have lower self-esteem and become more obsessed with weight loss, but the weird thing is that they don't lose their appetite.

In fact, they even have a more flourished appetite. During the late afternoons or evenings, they constantly look to binge on desserts and starches.

In one study done, bulimics were deprived of the single protein of tryptophan. As a response, their serotonin levels flattened and they binge even more -

ingesting and purging an average of 1000 calories each day.

Chronic depletion of plasma tryptophan may be one of those mechanisms where persistent dieting may lead to the development of further eating disorders in those who are vulnerable.

It is also important to note that most compulsive eaters don't vomit. They are able to keep it all down. However, dieting may further lower serotonin levels and cause the same wild cravings and self-hate that bulimics torture themselves with.

From here, it is clear that it is very easy for a dieter to develop an eating disorder. If you take the time to truly understand how many other critical brain and body chemicals are wiped out during dieting, you would have a sounder appreciation of the dangers of a low-caloric diet.

Chapter 6: The Process Of Recovery From Bulimia

If you realize that you have been living with bulimia, you would know exactly how scary it feels to be out of control. Knowing how you are harming your body simply adds to the fear of it.

However, don't worry. Change is possible regardless of how long you have been battling with this condition. You are able to break this habit of binging and purging and have a healthier attitude towards the food you eat and your body.

The steps towards recovery is very hard. It is very common to feel unsure about stopping your binging and purging habit even though it could be adverse. However, if you are thinking about getting help for bulimia already, you are taking a huge step forward.

The Bulimia Recovery Steps

- Firstly, **acknowledge that you have a problem**. You have been drummed into this idea that you your life would be greater and you would feel good if you lose weight. This is an idea that is drummed into your head when you are in control what you eat. Be clear that the very first step in the process of bulimia recovery. You would first need to acknowledge that your relationship to food is distorted and totally out of control.

- **Speak to somebody about the problem**. It could be very

uncomfortable to talk to someone about what you are going through, especially if you have kept your binge-eating a secret for a long period. You may be hesitant, ashamed or afraid about what other people think. Nevertheless, it is important to understand that you are not alone. Get someone who listens, somebody who would support you in your attempt to become better.

- **Be in the right environment**. Step back from places, activities or people who spark off the temptation to binge or purge. You may need to avoid looking too much of fitness or fashion magazines. You may need to spend less time with your other friends who are always dieting and talking about being thin. You should also keep away from weight loss websites which only encourage bulimia. You should also be very careful about recipe and cooking magazines or shows.

- **Seek professional help**. With the right advice and support from a trained eating specialist, you are better equipped to retrieve your good health. You would learn to eat normally again and develop healthier attitude towards your food and body.

Why You Should Choose NOT TO DIET

The treatment of bulimia has a higher chance of succeeding if you decide to stop dieting once and for all.

The moment you quit trying to restrict calories and follow strict dietary rules, you would no longer be overpowered with cravings and the desire for more food. By eating right, you would be able to break the binge and purge cycle; and achieve a common weight.

Treatment And Therapy For Bulimia

To break this cycle of binge-and-purge, it is especially important to seek professional help as soon as you can. You need to also follow it up with treatment to resolve the emotional problems that you have deep down. They may have induced the bulimia problem in the very first place.

As very often, the reason for bulimia lies in a poor body image and low self-esteem, therapy play a significant part of recovery. It is very common to feel isolated and ashamed by your pigging out and purging and therapists may assist with these feelings.

The most common treatment for bulimia is perhaps Cognitive Behavioural Therapy (CBT). CBT especially targets people who have unhealthy eating behaviours like bulimia or those who have unrealistic, damaging thoughts which push their punishing behaviour. The therapist would perform it and these are several things that you can expect during bulimia therapy:

1. **Stopping The Binge-And-Purge Cycle** - This primary phase of bulimia treatment focus on stopping this vicious cycle of overeating and purging. Over time, you are able to re-establish normal eating patterns. You would find out better on how to monitor your eating habits or to keep

away from situations which would trigger binges. Besides that, you would also cope with the tension better in a way which you don't require food. You would also learn to eat healthily to cut down on your unnecessary food cravings and battle the instinct to purge.

2. **Changing Unhealthy Thoughts** - The second phase of bulimia treatment is on identifying and altering those dysfunctional beliefs about your weight, body shape and dieting. You would explore the mental attitudes about your eating habits and rethink the belief that your self-esteem is based on how slim you are.

3. **Resolve Emotional Issues You Have** - The final phase of bulimia treatment would be on dealing with emotional problems which cause the eating disorder in the very first place. The therapy would focus on dealing with relationship problems, depression, tension, low self-esteem and feeling of loneliness.

When you have bulimia, it may feel like you can't escape from your eating disorder. Nevertheless, keep in mind that recovery is always within your grasp. With the proper treatment, support from loved one and self-help methods; you would be able to overpower this bulimia condition and gain more self-assurance.

Final Notes On Bulimia

If you have this suspicion that your friend or loved ones have bulimia, you would need to talk to them about your problem. He or she may deny that you have this overeating and purging problem, but there is a higher possibility that he or she would receive with open arms the chance to be more open up his or her battle.

Regardless, bulimia can never be pushed aside as the person's physical and emotional health is at stake. It is very terrible to know that someone you love who is so young may be binging and purging. However, you need to know that you can never force someone with an eating disorder to modify their behaviour and you won't be able to do all the work in the process of recovery for another person.

But you can still provide all the encouragement, compassion and support throughout the treatment procedure.

If you have a loved one with bulimia, you should provide all the support and compassion. Be clear that the individual may even get defensive or mad. However, if he or she doesn't open up, listen to what they have to say without any judgment and show that you care.

You should keep away from insulting them or using other psychological remarks which may harm them. Since bulimia is a condition which is often caused and made worse by tension, low self-esteem and shame; negativity would only bring more problems.

Besides that, you should also set a great example. You should eat healthily and exercise well. You should also stop talking too much about your body or anyone else.

You should also be clear to set boundaries. When you are a parent or friends, there isn't much you can do to fix your loved one's bulimia problem. The individual would need to move forward himself.

Besides that, always understand the value of professional therapy. The advice which you get from counsellors is always better. Dealing with eating disorder is difficult, but it can be easy if you have professional help.

In conclusion, bulimia is a condition which is difficult without knowing the right thing. Believe in yourself and your ability to fix yourself from this condition. Good luck!

Resource 1 - Cure Bulimia Using The Advances In Technology

Discover how scientific research unlocked the key to lifelong recovery from bulimia...

This is an amazing guide that shows you how you could use amazing SCIENTIFIC RESEARCH to cure bulimia ONCE AND FOR ALL.

4 Reasons Why The Bulimia Help Method Works When Other Treatments Don't

- *We help you resolve the core problem of food restriction (surprisingly most treatment programs tend to gloss over this).*

- *It's simple and easy for you to understand and follow (so you don't get confused, lost or fed up).*

- *You are guided step-by-step along the way so you always know what to expect and what to do next.*

- *You are supported by the webs largest bulimia community (they understand exactly what you are going through).*

Get it now from...

http://bulimiahelp.wellbeingvalley.com/

Resource 2 - The Bulimia Recovery Program

This is another amazing and simple method of bulimia recovery. It is only based on three simple BUT HIGHLY EFFECTIVE STEPS:

(1) Structured Eating

(2) Self-Kindness

(3) Neuroplasticity

This is perhaps the most incredible guide, together with an invaluable bulimia recovery community. Find out more from:-

http://overcomebulimia.wellbeingvalley.com/

www.ingramcontent.com/pod-product-compliance
Lightning Source LLC
Chambersburg PA
CBHW070555290526

45790CB00002B/701